The Weight Pop Off Method:
Rhymes For Weight Pop Off Times

The Weight Pop Off Method:
Rhymes For Weight Pop Off Times

A Book To Help You Gain A Better Look

The Weight Pop Off Method:
Rhymes For Weight Pop Off Times

Nicholas Hester, PhD

Edited by Nikki Baldwin

Nicholas Hester
2018

First Printing: 2018

ISBN: 978-1-387-94956-4

Contents

Introduction

It might just take a little rhyme

To bring about weight pop off time

Because you might need to hear things in a different way

For weight loss motivation to remain high all day

Well, that is just what this book is for

For you to stay focused & use all that you have in store

The rhymes will always remain in your head

And your motivation & good behaviors will spread

So read the rhymes now & your bad habits will drop off

Because I know you are ready, for weight to POP OFF!

THE RHYMES

"Excuses Are No More"

Those silly excuses won't fly anymore

Because a healthy lifestyle, you will no longer ignore

It's never too late in your life

To make better decisions with the fork & knife

You are never too tired to win

That's just laziness, trying to take over again

You can't use the "wait until tomorrow" excuse

Because that's just downright body abuse

It's not alright to skip healthiness "just today"

That attitude, will make your dream body hopes fade away

Do you complain about not having enough time in the day?

Well newsflash, the fit life doesn't have to take hours a day

You don't have the excuse of not knowing what to do

You have "The Weight Pop Off Method" ready to help you

So before you form an excuse with your lips

Think more about your health, and start moving your hips!

"Pop Off That Weight"

It's time for you to pop off those pounds

Which will definitely feel, as good as that sounds

The "Weight Pop Off Method" lets you take control of your head

To make the decisions, that will allow your good habits to spread

The method calls for you to plan & evaluate each week

And to stay consistent, to quickly reach your peak

The method calls for you to weekly find

Foods & workouts, that will keep you from a decline

The method describes how you can make adjustments to do better

So that you will have a body, deserving of a newsletter

The method describes different fitness activities

Which will lead you to, the weight loss festivities

The method calls for you to try healthier options of foods you like

Which will allow you to send, unhealthy foods on a permanent hike

From now on, following the method is what you will do

Which will leave you surprised, at how fast the weight flies off you!

"Ready In All Ways"

Are you ready to pop off that weight?

Are you ready to have a fantastic body as your fate?

If you are ready, then you must set a goal

One you must remember, when stress starts to take a toll

You should be ready to change your whole lifestyle

Probably to doing those things, you haven't done in a while

From now on, there is nothing that can hold you back

Therefore it's totally on you, to make sure that you stay on track

But you will get to reap the rewards in every way

Because you will get smarter, plus give a supreme effort everyday

You will not worry about a slip or a fall

Because you will have the confidence, to overcome it all

So hopefully your answer to being ready is "yes"

That way you can be happy, and deserving of ultimate success!

"The Winning Goal"

Winning starts by defining your specific goal

One that will help get you out, of the overweight hole

For most, the obvious goal is to lose weight

But you have to answer "how much", to have a greater fate

Put an amount of pounds to lose per month and per week

For the best chance to stay focused, and remain at your peak

Make sure that your goal is something realistic

So that you won't quit early, or have your mind go ballistic

Include goals that focus on improving your health & well-being

Because this method improves the body, and is also mind-freeing

Ultimately, the goals you set will be the reason why

You run a little more, or put down that slice of pie

Just make sure that your goals mean the absolute world to you

To have a better chance, of having great weight loss come true!

"Activation Of Your Motivation"

The goal is set, now you have to activate

Well, if you really want to drop that weight

Let's start with your mental game & thought process

You have to believe, that you CAN lead yourself to success

You have to know that you CAN do everything it will take

Or you will go back down, the unhealthy road that you hate

Next, you need to make sure some items or people get eliminated

Especially the ones, that leave you feeling humiliated

Thus, get rid of what you need & take a firm stance

For you to see your fitness goal stand its best chance

So get ready to formulate your great plan

Because you are now mentally ready, and also fully understand

That with your all, you have to move to the stage of activation

And you undoubtedly know, there is no more time for hesitation!

"Determination For Your Elevation"

Losing your fitness battle is taking its toll

But only because, your mind has yet to take control

Your current health may have you upset & annoyed

Or feeling as if, your body looks destroyed

But those feelings are seriously about to stop

Because your mind is about to 100% Pop-

Off with raised motivation & full determination

To reach a body, that will look good on your next vacation

Thus, it starts now & not any other day later

That you train your mindset, to be significantly greater

So that you can fend off each pessimistic & negative thought

About how you will lose, before you have even fought

Just use all that "The Weight Pop Off Method" does teach

And you will soon be able, to take your dream body to the beach!

"To Late To Wait"

People keep telling you that it is too late

For you to lose, an amount of weight that will fascinate

Maybe you have even said this to yourself

Which you know is unfavorable, to your own eyes & your health

Instead of saying too late, say that you are long overdue

And then say you are ready, to earn a new body for you

Even if age-wise you are starting a little later

You are still going to prove, to each & every doubting hater

That you are on the fitness attack

And you won't let your age, ever hold you back

So now the only thing that is keeping you from your win

Is to say that it's not too late, for you to begin!

"Stand & Then Stand Some More"

It's time to take an unwavering stand

And vow to never depart, from your personal plan

Once you decide to take this stand

You will find, that you are always in command

To lose weight, you must always remember the word "stand"

Because it will help you, obtain a weight loss that is grand

Stand means to get off the couch, and up on to your feet

So you will put down that treat, and never have to face defeat

Sometimes you should stand when you eat

Because we all eat more, when eating from a seat

Understand, that from henceforth you are definitely in a fight

So you will need to stand up, for treating your body right

Because there are many temptations that you will need to withstand

But you DO have the strength, to reach your weight loss dreamland!

"Feel It All"

It's time to go ahead & be real

And admit to yourself how you feel

You need to admit those feelings of disgust

About how you are feeling overly fat & robust

Become angry with how you made it to your current shape

But also understand, why you have those feelings of hate

Because it is these feelings of depressing frustration

That will give you, the most appropriate motivation

To make sure that your unhealthy habits go away

Leaving the desired YOU, here to rewardingly stay

It's funny how these negative feelings are something that could

Lead you to a body size, that feels so extremely good

So keep those negative feelings in mind

To stay locked in, on your "Weight Pop Off Method" grind!

"For Who & For What Though?"

Who & what are you doing this for?

Is this just for you, or maybe for something more?

Maybe it's to impress your loved ones or kids

By showing them, the proper way to live

It most certainly should be to improve your health

So one answer, is most certainly for yourself

But your purpose should also be for something more

So you stay motivated, to give all the energy you have in store

Maybe the purpose is for the stress relief benefit

So you won't explode, or be caught throwing a fit

Maybe the purpose is to look like more of an attraction

To certain people, from which you want a favorable reaction

Maybe the purpose is to get back at people that poked fun of you

For them to be shocked, at your weight loss breakthrough

Maybe the purpose is for some type of event

So you can look good enough, to be happy you went

Just think of several reasons why you want to get out of your hole

Because each one will push you, closer to your desired weight goal!

"A Simple Choice"

Would you not trade your unhealthy pleasure

To gain significant weight loss as your treasure?

Will you not give a little more of your time

To gain a body that you consider sublime?

Are you not willing to put down the spoon & the fork

To try something you know will clearly work?

Can you not get yourself off the couch

To help rid yourself of that pouch?

Will you not get rid of each & every excuse

To stop committing unwanted body abuse?

Will you not make sure that you have the effort to give

For you to stay healthy each day that you live?

Will you not avoid stopping for fatty fast food

To avoid having overweight depression as your mood?

Will you not avoid those people that trigger

You to do all the unhealthy things that make you bigger?

So just make sure that you are willing to do

Everything necessary, to gain the spectacular & thin version of you!

"No Stopping, Just Winning"

Who said that you could be stopped?

Whoever said it, needs to be popped

Because no one gets a say in what you can do

Whether you will be stopped, falls directly upon you

Just let people continue to hate & have their doubt

It won't stop you, from bringing your weight loss about

People will try to stop you from reaching your best

But by the end of your journey, they will be shockingly impressed

Now, there are some habits that need to be stopped

For your weight loss dreams not to be popped

You know of those habits with which you struggle

And you also know what to do, to get rid of that trouble

Just make sure that your bad habits are dropped

So your weight loss dreams, won't flop or ever be stopped!

"Demand A Good Plan"

Your weight loss could be the greatest in the land

But first, you must come up with a specialized plan

A plan that will keep you steadily motivated

Until the day, you can be joyously congratulated

The plan must allow for you to MAKE the time

To remain consistent, while on your fitness grind

The plan must include how you can keep going all out

Even during those times, when you are having some doubt

The plan must include the days that will be the most intense

As well as include, when rest days will make the most sense

For the most part, you must stick to your plan

But some things will happen, that are just out of your command

Those happenings will not be an excuse for you to give up

They just mean your plan needs adjusting, to keep moving on up

If you have a great plan, then your results will show

If not, then this goal is something that you surely will blow

So get started now on planning for your entire week

And you soon will reach, every single goal that you seek!

"It's Fun To Lose Weight"

Participating in fitness can certainly be fun

Fun enough, to ensure that you get the job done

There are so many activities that you can do

Which are fun enough, to make you want to push through

The activities can be inside or out

Just be sure to have enough space, to let your energy out

Finding a favorite fun activity or two

Will help you lose pounds, and more than just a few

The fun activities will help in relieving any stress

With the added bonus, of bringing you weight loss progress

With so many fun fitness activities to choose

There is absolutely no excuse, for you to lose

So get out there & try something new

And you will see how fun & rewarding, fitness can be for you!

"Not Here For Fear"

Going after this goal might have you afraid

But by the end, you will see how wonderfully you are made

It is okay to have some health-related fears

Like the feeling you will have, from missing workouts with peers

Another healthy fear is to worry about your health

Which is a fear, that will help you reach the fit-life with stealth

Maybe you have a fear of your current body aches & pains

Well those could be minimized, if you work out & train

There is no need to be afraid because of your age

Age just helps you know, the discipline you need at this stage

Your fear should be motivating & not sad

Motivating enough, to gain the best body you've ever had

Thus, the main reason that you should not be afraid to reach your goal

Is because you are not scared, and you have outright control!

"Eat For The Win"

Tell me again why you won't put down that food?

Especially when it leads, to your hopes becoming screwed

Is it worth it just to have that taste?

Even though your goals & hopes will go to waste

Will you continue to make a daily fast food stop?

When you know that is why, your weight will not drop

It's past due time, for you to make a new plan for how to eat

So that your weight loss dreams, do not end in defeat

Your plan should start with throwing or giving away that stuff

That always leaves your body, looking & feeling so rough

Then it's time to choose some much healthier options

That will still be tasty, with the properly made concoctions

A simple tip is to add more daily fruit

Which can be the perfect sweet-snack substitute

An additional key to winning, is to start meal prepping

Which will ensure, that in the right direction you are stepping

Another key is to minimize time around an unhealthy friend

Because they could care less, if your goal comes to a crashing end

So try not to always reach for an unhealthy treat

And a hot body will be your reward, which is a way better treat!

"Don't Be Dumb From Your Momentum"

Be sure to watch out for the momentum curse

It can make you slack off, to a point where you have never felt worse

It happens when you start to do well & succeed

But get big-headed, and stop doing everything you need

Then all of sudden you take a look down at the scale

And you find that you are on the way, to an epic fitness fail

To avoid this, plan for the days & times that you will slack

And also have a plan, that describes how you can jump right back

Into those habits that ensure your success will continue to come

Or you will be left, feeling irresponsible & dumb

But if you evaluate daily whether you are doing what you should

Then the momentum curse, won't be able to curse you real good

So yes, be happy with each bit of success

But make sure that each bit, pushes you to keep giving your best!

"Use All Of The Hate"

They don't know what you can do

 So their negativity shouldn't get to you

What they think doesn't even matter

Just know that you WILL stop getting fatter

That might sound funny, but it is definitely true

Because weight loss, is about to come raining down upon you

Their unwanted hatred, harsh words, & doubt

Are just the push you need, to MAKE your body change come about

Because of them, you will have all the needed drive

For your journey to leave you feeling happy, successful, & alive

So start to think about how amazing it will feel

To show off a body, that has plenty of sex appeal

But first, you have to take all the hateful voices

And use them as motivation, for you to make healthy choices

And in the end, you will know that it was partially because of them

That you became confident, sexy, slender, & slim!

"Keep On Looking At Them"

Do you see those fit people over there?

It's okay, they make everybody want to stare

You can have a little hatred for them if you want

Just know, that they are giving the effort that you won't

From now on, your feelings for them will change

Because visions of them, will spark your successful body exchange

Though now your body might seem far from ideal

Their looks will motivate you, to be successful at each meal

Getting to how they look may take a little time

But thoughts of their habits, will help you create your own shine

So the next time you are about to eat unhealthily or be lazy

Think about what they would do, so you won't do something crazy

Now from here on out, turn your jealous feelings into motivation

And you will soon be on your way, to an amazing body creation!

"From Busy To Getting Busy"

Being too busy is not an acceptable excuse

That's just another example of committing body abuse

We all have the same amount of time in each day

So you decide, if you want to let your time waste away

You are not too busy to put one foot in front of the other

Or to get up off the couch, or from underneath the cover

You have not been too busy to go get unhealthy food with friends

Or to eat those unhealthy comfort foods by the bins

You make excuses to avoid putting in an effort that will work

But those excuses have left you, feeling like an overweight jerk

Now is the time to stop excusing yourself from success

And to start excusing yourself, from things that hinder your progress

Because you do have the time to make a better choice at your meal

And to move just a little more, no matter how lazy you feel

You do have the time, just not a bit of time to lose

So make sure that this time, it's good behaviors that you choose!

"Help For The Real You"

Only you can hold yourself accountable

For doing something, that might seem insurmountable

But get at least one person that can help keep you on track

A person to help make sure, you don't keep falling back

It has to be someone you can definitely trust

Someone that hopes, your weight loss dreams don't end in a bust

This person could be a family member or friend

And it would really help, to have similar fitness goals as them

This person could be a personal trainer or coach

Who could ensure, that you have the right techniques & approach

They will help you get into the health & physique that you want

Plus far, far away, from those insulting taunts

They should push you & always be honest

So that you will put forth, your best effort upon this

Just know that this will be a fight & a journey

So this person should be willing to fight for you like an attorney

So even though it is your new body to win

You will get there faster, with the help of a friend!

"The Dipping Sauce"

You could be a champion of weight loss

By simply changing your dipping sauce

The current foods you eat might be healthy & all

But those sauces & dressings, could be the reason that you fall

It seems harmless to dip your food into this or to that

But be aware, that those dips could be making you fat

To fix, try limiting the amount of sauce that you use

Or make sure, that it is a healthier option that you choose

Just by reading the contents on the sauce label

You will know which sauces, should be removed from the table

There are many healthier options for you to still enjoy the flavor

Which will do wonders, for working in your weight pop off favor

Choosing wisely can lower the calories, fat, & sodium in your meal

As well as be the key to success, in your whole weight loss ordeal!

"Eat How Often?"

You must know when you should eat

Because waiting too long, could bring your goals to defeat

It is important to portion size your food & eat often

So that your cravings, for unhealthy & big meals will soften

This will require you to plan for the foods you will consume

And sticking to that plan, will keep you far away from doom

It's hard to pinpoint the exact times that you can feed

So you need to also plan, for the types of snacks you may need

If your plan includes a typical schedule of when & what you will eat

You will have this weight loss journey halfway complete

Then it is up to you to stay the course

And keep yourself away, from every temptational source

But that will be easy by eating frequently & only what you planned

So soon you will see weight popping off, just as fast as it can!

"Emotional Goodness"

On those days when you feel down

Do you find yourself just sitting around?

Or eating unhealthy food by the pound?

Well no more of that emotional unhealthy eating

Because that just adds, to the stress of any emotional beating

Each time you reach for an unhealthy bag

It will contribute to making your body sag

And that is not stated just to be rude

It's just what you need to hear, to stay in a weight pop off mood

Plus, you see what has happened from being out of shape

And from eating unhealthy foods, no matter the size or the shape

From now on, if emotions don't cause you to be unhealthy

Then the people who laughed at you, will soon be looking crazy

Because once you are able to control your eating with every emotion

You will have the ingredient, for your successful weight loss potion!

"Adjust Is A Must"

One thing that is a must

Is that you, must learn how to adjust

You first must adjust to a new positive mindset

So that you will not stop, until your goals have been met

Getting adjusted to your new habits will only take a week or two

Which is definitely worth it, to become a skinnier version of you

Eventually you will have to adjust the workouts that you do

Because your body will adapt, to any fitness routine chosen for you

You will need to adjust in activity, intensity, & duration

To continue to feel that weight loss sensation

You will also need to adjust your diet from time to time

To different healthy foods, during your appointed meal times

Conquering all the ways you need to adjust

Will keep you from ending up, as a disappointing weight loss bust

So if you really want to stop those weight-referenced insults

Adjustments will be needed, for satisfying & lasting results!

"Decide To Be A Great Decision Maker"

Every good decision you make will be pleasing

And each positive action helps, for weight loss goal seizing

Every extra step that you take

Is needed, because you ate that extra slice of cake

Each time that you decide to hit the gym

Will move you closer to a body, that's amazingly slim & trim

Each time you decide to do a weekly meal prep

Will be a week away, from the fast food doorstep

Every time you decide to pass on desert

Will help you get into those jeans, or into that skirt

Each time you decide to put down the sauce or the jelly

Will help with getting rid of your unwanted potbelly

Each time you decide to show your healthy lifestyle dedication

Your body will unveil its stunning appreciation

And when everything mentioned becomes a habit

Your goal will be so close, that you can reach out & grab it!

"One Is Your Number"

Everyone knows that we are supposed to portion size

But instead we add extra food, that shows up in our thighs

The key to portion sizing is to remember the number one

And associate that, with eating only "one" & be done

If you can stick to having just one plate

Then you will reach your goals, by your desired date

If you can limit yourself to just one bowl

It will make you feel good, deep down in your soul

If you can keep each of your servings to just one

Your weight loss efforts, will never come undone

If you can change one bad eating habit a week

You will be rewarded, with the weight loss goal that you seek

So when you finally get this number of "one" down

You soon will be living a life, of not having to lose another pound!

"Laugh Your Way To Weight Loss"

People may have laughed at your body size & weight

But now, laughter will become an important weight loss trait

The more that you can incorporate humor

Will help the weight pop off even sooner

Your weight loss journey will have times of stress

But humor is one of the ways, to alleviate stress best

Laugh at how badly you treated your body in the past

Because now you know, that the bad treatment has passed

Find something that will make you laugh at night

And you will wake up feeling energized, and also full of delight

Your workout time on the treadmill will go by really fast

While you watch a funny show, on your telecast

Spend some time daily, joking with a family member or friend

And you will feel good enough, to work for your weight loss win

The bottom line is that humor will make you feel pleasant

Which is the needed feel, to obtain weight loss as your present!

"The Vision To Avoid a Collision"

If weight loss is where you will succeed

Then visualization, is a skill you will need

You need to visualize with each & every sense

For the "Weight Pop Off Method", to truly commence

You need to see visions of yourself in your desired figure

To push yourself, to stop getting bigger

Visualize all the welcomed praises you will hear

If you work hard enough, to make your new body appear

Visualize being able to avoid those tempting smells

And see yourself eating healthy, when you hear the dinner bells

Visualize touching your body, and it feeling fit & hard

Because being lazy, is something you will now be able to discard

Visualize how good weight loss success will taste

Then get started, because you have no more time to waste!

"Defeat Your Cheat"

It's not alright to slack off & cheat

If you have not been watching what you eat

Or if you have not been moving your lazy feet

Sure you can cheat a little & still win

But not just as soon, as your weight loss efforts begin

Cheating should only come if you deserve

Not something, that you consistently serve

A cheat meal, or a non-workout day needs to be planned

If you want to witness, weight loss happen first-hand

Be sure to schedule your cheats scarcely though

So that your weight loss results, will continue to grow

And yes, everyone makes a mistake once in a while

Just don't let them happen, too often in your new lifestyle

So if you want to be rewarded with a cheat day

Then you need to stay focused, on what you really want to weigh!

ABOUT THE AUTHOR

Nicholas Hester, PhD has a life goal of helping people succeed and feel happy about themselves in every aspect of life. He is the author of "The Weight Pop Off Method" series, which allows individuals to take control of their fitness and eating habits to reach their weight loss and body image goals. He is the author of the "Pop Into Success" series, which gives inspiring words to help people realize career, fitness, athletic, and student success. He is the author of the "Stop Stopping Your Unstoppableness" series, in which words and quotes are given to help individuals evaluate their lives and get motivated to succeed. Lastly, he is the author of the "Gaining Your ExtrAbility" series, which helps individuals to use all they have to take themselves to an astonishing level of success.

Nicholas Hester has a Doctor of Philosophy degree in Exercise and Sport Psychology. He works at a University where he inspires students to do their best and teaches several workshops on personal and social development. He also works as a personal trainer and is a Certified Strength and Conditioning Specialist. Lastly, he is a motivational speaker that inspires people to find it in themselves to work hard and become the person that they want to be.

www.ingramcontent.com/pod-product-compliance
Lightning Source LLC
Chambersburg PA
CBHW050351290526
45785CB00006B/2730